The 5:2 Diet:
Single-Serving
Vegetarian Recipes

Belinda Price

ISBN:1484128044
ISBN-13: 978-1484128046

Disclaimer:

I have checked all the details of this book several times to ensure it is as accurate as possible. If any errors have escaped my notice I cannot accept responsibility, though I apologise for the unlikely occurrence of any inconvenience caused.

CONTENTS

Index of Recipes (page numbers in brackets)

Breakfasts

Lunches

Summer Salad: 83 calories (48)
Spicy Cauliflower: 140 calories (51)
Mediterranean Vegetable Roast: 91 calories (54)
Cauliflower Soup: 87 calories (57)
Sweet & Sour Salad: 87 calories (60)
Coleslaw: 79 calories (63)
Quick Minestrone Soup: 197 calories (66)
Carrot and Cumin Soup: 108 calories (69)
Yoghurt Waldorf Salad: 233 calories (72)

Suppers

Cauliflower Bake: 157 calories (16)
Stir Fry Bok Choy: 236 calories (19)
Cheese & Onion Frittata: 195 calories (22)
Scrambled Egg with Chives: 190 calories (25)
Spinach & Onion Omelette: 184 calories (28)
Lemon and Parsley Couscous: 249 calories (31)
Feta Tortilla Wrap: 267 calories (34)
Vegetable Broth: 236 calories (37)
Chinese Ginger Vegetables: 213 calories (40)
Carrot & Lentil Soup: 237 calories (43)
Stuffed Pepper: 303 calories (46)
Twirly Pasta,Tomatoes, Spinach & Cheese: 339 calories (49)
Basil & Tomato Scrambled Eggs: 195 calories (52)
Spaghetti with Courgette (Zucchini) & Onion: 342 calories (55)
Mixed Roast Vegetables with Pasta: 313 calories (58)
Vegetable Goulash: 313 calories (61)
Chinese Ginger Vegetables: 225 calories (64)
Pasta with Tomato Sauce: 190 calories (67)
Tofu and Quinoa: 240 calories (70)
Spiced Lentil Stew: 187 calories (73)

The 5:2 Diet Explained

The 5:2 Diet simply defined:

This diet is sometimes known as the Fasting Diet, the Intermittent Fasting Diet or the Fasting and Feasting Diet. They all come down to the same principle, though I prefer to drop the word "fasting" as it can convey a misleading (and perhaps off-putting) impression.

- You choose *any* two days per week you wish and cut the total number of calories consumed on those days to a quarter of the recommended daily amount. So if you are female you can eat 500 and if you are male it's 600 calories for each of those days. You can change those days around as you wish each week to fit in with your social calendar. The only rule to this is that the days are not consecutive.

- It is completely up to you whether to skip breakfast and/or lunch, reserving all or most of your calories for your evening meal; or to consume the bulk of your day's calories for breakfast. Alternatively, you can spread your calories to allow for three meals on your low-calorie days. This book is designed for this last option, though you can, if you wish, simply select one or two recipes from any day and supplement your intake with drinks or your own recipe to add up to your daily allowance. You have ***total control*** over the way you do the 5:2 diet.

- No food as such is banned from your two low calorie days so long as it doesn't exceed the target number of calories.

- On the other five days of your week you can please yourself what you eat or drink. Chocolate, wine, cakes... all

3

these treats are permitted, although it makes good sense to consume them in moderation. I know of no other diet that is as flexible about food.

- On the 5:2 diet no food is classed as a "sin", allowed only in small amounts or completely forbidden.

*

Impressive ways in which this novel way of eating could change your life forever:

- Your weight loss is guaranteed if you stick to the principles outlined within these pages. This benefit will undoubtedly be the first to become apparent. You can be confident that you are on the path to banishing those unwanted pounds of fat forever! In itself this is sufficiently rewarding to encourage you to carry on even before you reap the other benefits.

- You will ultimately feel more energised.

- Exercising will become easier as you will have less weight to carry around.

- Your appetite on the five "normal" days of eating will gradually decrease as your stomach shrinks and you feel less need for large amounts of food.

- It will quite possibly prevent the mental deterioration that we are all prone to develop with age – Alzheimer's disease, dementia, Parkinson's disease... An enormous amount of research has been done over several years, with rodents, to back up this claim. And, even if you are not a rodent results are promising; the increasing numbers of human studies substantiate the findings with animals.

- Just two days each week involving lowered calorie intake can make all the difference to how healthily we live our lives. It could also dramatically increase our longevity. This is because the level of a growth hormone called the IGF1 hormone, which tends to be produced in large amounts as we age, is automatically lowered when we calorie restrict. This reduction triggers the body into repairing existing damaged cells rather than focus on new cell manufacture. Once this occurs, harm that may have been done to your body over the years can, in this marvellous work of reparation, actually begin to reverse the damage done to your body in the past, giving you renewed hope for a healthier and hopefully, happier future!

- Hunger appears to make the brain more alert, though in the early weeks of the diet you will probably experience short-lived hunger pangs until your body adjusts. These can easily be soothed with plenty of calorie- free cold drinks of health-giving water and/or hot, non-calorie drinks such as black or green tea. So your memory power should improve and your ability to think sharpen considerably.

- Eating the 5:2 way can normalise blood sugar, avoiding the danger of type 2 diabetes, which is usually associated with obesity in adulthood.

- Cholesterol levels can be lowered, thereby significantly diminishing the risks of developing heart disease.

- Research strongly suggests that keeping to the 5:2 diet plan can play an important role in preventing development of various cancers and other serious diseases. Once again, human research in this area, though not yet extensive, supports the outcomes of animal studies.

*

We could well be on the brink of an exciting breakthrough in this aspect of research. Already we are aware of a group of approximately three hundred people in the world who have what is termed 'Laron's Syndrome'. These individuals are born without the growth-related IGF1 hormone and grow to less than four feet as adults. So, not having the hormone is a disadvantage when they are young. However, despite their shortness of height they all live long, reasonably healthy lives without suffering from the diseases we usually associate with aging. Indeed, were it not for the fact the some of them drink alcohol excessively and smoke, who knows how much longer they might live?

To summarise: by following the 5:2 diet it would seem that we stand a far better than average chance of living longer, active, disease-free lives. Who could realistically ask for more, except perhaps to win the lottery...

Now you are equipped with all the important basic facts you need to know to begin the 5:2 diet.

To help you on your way, this book contains twenty each of recipes for vegetarian breakfasts, lunches and suppers, complete with calorie counts at the start of each meal and the total for each day. A man's extra 100 calorie allowance can easily be topped up, using these recipes, with an added portion of vegetables (vegetables being on the whole low calorie means he could have a reasonably generous portion) or a low calorie snack. A few of the meals I have included can simply be doubled in quantity.

*

Important Note

> *It is essential to mention at this point that there are a few groups of people for whom this diet is definitely unsuitable. They are:*

- *Pregnant or breastfeeding women*
- *Children*
- *Diabetics*
- *Anyone with a history of eating disorders*

However, anyone who has a health condition for which they are being treated by their GP should discuss the wisdom, or not, of proceeding with this or any other diet.

My Personal Experience

The 5:2 diet is not a really hard diet to stick to. Eight months on, I can state this with absolute assurance and conviction. Yet, before beginning the 5:2 diet, I had never stayed on *any* diet for more than a few weeks, at the very most. Every one I came across involved a strong dose of sustained willpower. It had taken me many years to quit smoking and I was not prepared to undertake anything that was equally difficult. So, after searching for several years for *the* diet that could suit my love of food and lack of commitment, I was fast reaching the conclusion that there was, in fact, no such diet – until the 5:2 hit the scene.

Although I already possessed a blender I treated myself to a juicer and citrus squeezer to make life that much easier. And I mustered up every bit of enthusiasm I could, determined to apply myself single-mindedly to my first day of calorie restricting. After a weekend of my usual comfort eating, I began.

When I first started, though, I was more than a little concerned that 500 calories would consist of far too little to fill me up for a day. I was slightly horrified when I found out that the baked potato with cheese and baked beans I was planning for my evening meal on the first day totalled a massive 532 calories – more than my allotted allowance for the entire day! Additionally, when I totted up the number of calories I had already consumed by suppertime, it came to 320, even though I thought I had been pretty meagre in my choice – a glass of orange juice and a slice of wholemeal bread spread with peanut butter for breakfast and only a pear for lunch.

Perhaps this diet, that so many people I knew were enthusing about, was not for me. Maybe, I would just have to resign myself to being five stone overweight, I thought unhappily. But my husband's promise of a summer holiday in the South of France the following year, to celebrate our fifteenth wedding anniversary, spurred me on. I wanted so much to fit comfortably into that seat on the plane and not attract stares as I ventured onto the beach in my swimming costume.

I decided that I would keep going with this diet for a month and if, by then, I was finding it unbearably hard I would abandon it and wait for the next new diet to come along.

I began to plan my two low calorie days carefully in advance, working out the calorie content of each recipe I used. The problem was that, although my husband is also a vegetarian, he had no intention of doing this diet with me. To be honest, he's not overweight and he said he wasn't going to start dieting in the hope of living a few years longer; he also told me that I looked beautiful, whatever my size. Despite his compliment, I sat down and added my doctor's recent stern warning - that I was on track to develop diabetes if I did not cut down on the amount I ate - to my list of incentives to get started. I would go it alone.

During the first few weeks I have to admit that I hit a number of obstacles, quite apart from what food to put on my plate on a calorie restricted day.

Initially, I was missing meals, usually breakfast, and feeling totally lacking in energy. So I began to work on having three daily as I had been used to. This is, after all, not meant to be a starvation diet and eating my usual number of meals made the whole experience feel more familiar to me.

As my low calorie day wore on I found I began to get a headache. When I mentioned this to one of my friends who started the diet around the same time I did, she suggested drinking a glass of water before each meal and a few more glasses than I normally did during the day; this seemed to do the trick and the energy dips stopped also .

Another problem was that, although I knew it was a good idea to increase my fluid intake, I wasn't sure, at first, what I could drink throughout the day, other than water, without adding to the calories. So I did a bit of research and compiled a list of calorie-free drinks to choose from, (you'll find it at the beginning of the next section).

If I got to the end of one of my two days feeling tired and/or a bit unsure whether I had the stamina to continue with this diet, I would have an early night and console myself with the thought that the next day I could eat whatever I wished.

Oddly enough though, I found after the first couple of weeks that I no longer had the voracious craving for food I've had for years. I would prepare a meal, on my 'normal' days, only to find I couldn't eat more than half of it. This reduction in appetite was an unexpected but welcome bonus, though it's quite logical if I'd stopped to think about it.

As the weeks turned into months I encountered a further effect of my altered style of eating: my size 20 clothes were ill fitting and unflattering. Time I would once have spent snacking on calorie laden snacks got used up browsing clothes shops for some new, more attractive items of clothing. Busying myself on my low calorie days was, for me, an important way to cope whilst following my new eating patterns. I enjoy cooking and focused far more on shopping for ingredients and making my meals than I had done previously. Sometimes, when a hunger pang struck (and they did quite often in those early weeks) I would distract myself with my watercolours, immerse myself in a good book or concentrate on writing. And, any time I saw someone eating a cream cake or an ice cream, I would remind myself that I only had to wait until my twenty-four hours were up to indulge if I felt so inclined. That way I did not feel I was missing out.

Instead of adding calorie–laden sugar to a recipe I sometimes substituted stevia, a totally natural plant extract with zero calories (a third of a teaspoon is equivalent to a full teaspoon of granulated sugar). Surprisingly, however, my cravings for sweet foods have decreased dramatically.

A further couple of notes on substitution – I find that liquid egg white can sometimes be an excellent alternative to eggs; besides being only 15 calories instead of 55 where a small egg might be used, it is much lower in cholesterol.

And I found that having a one calorie oil spray in stock is especially useful, particularly when you realise that a tablespoon of olive oil is 120 calories.

My weight loss has been slow but steady and I find it a lot easier to move around and so do more exercise than before I started this diet. I actually feel energetic, a word I never dreamed I would ever use with reference to myself. I look forward to my low calorie days and they never interfere with my social life – any time I go out to eat I simply swap the days around, if necessary, for that week. In fact, I rarely keep to the same two days, preferring to remain completely flexible about my weekly scheduling. And I have noticed an improvement in my mood, perhaps, in no small part, because I am now within healthy weight limits and physically lighter.

I am still enjoying the 5:2 diet, still finding it rewarding (not least the prospect of this slimmer, more energetic me walking along the beach in Cannes in August) and have every intention of continuing indefinitely. It's a lifestyle choice that I am glad I made. I was amazed, after only eight months, when I jumped on the scales for my weekly weigh-in, to discover that I had achieved my goal – I was five stone lighter than when I began the diet! It was a great moment. If you had asked me a year ago if I thought it was possible I would have laughed or groaned, or both. I immediately rang two of my friends, who are also on the 5:2 diet, with the good news. The three of us have cajoled, encouraged and praised each other along the way.

So finally, here it is the diet that suits me and I'm sure will suit you.

My journey, so far, has inspired me to write this book. If I can do this diet, you can too!

Calorie-Free Drinks (or almost!)

The following is a list of drinks that are either completely calorie free or contain no more than a couple of calories each. This list is obviously not exhaustive, but will at least provide you with a few ideas for drinks for your 2 calorie restricted days.

Water (tap or bottled)

Sparkling water

Diet cola

Diet soda

Iced tea

Black tea

Green tea

Earl Grey tea

Rooibos tea (Red Bush)

Vast variety of fruit teas / fruit infusions (1-3 calories)

You can make your own flavoured water by taking a large jug of cold water and adding slices of low calorie fruit or vegetables, such as cucumber, lemons or strawberries, or herbs, such as mint or basil. These are virtually calorie-free drinks.

Menus

Day 1: 496 calories

Breakfast

Poached Eggs with Mushrooms: 135 calories

> 1 slice wholemeal bread
> 1 small egg
> 1 drop of vinegar
> Pinch of salt
> 56g (2 oz) button mushrooms, wiped clean with a damp paper towel
> 1- cal vegetable oil spray

Bring to the boil a half-filled medium saucepan of salted water.

Put a slice of toast into a toaster

Spray a frying pan with 4 sprays of 1-cal oil and heat gently

Break the egg into a cup and add a drop of vinegar (this helps the egg to keep its shape in the pan).

Whisk or stir the boiling water vigorously to make it swirl and drop the egg into the middle.

Reduce the heat to low and cook for about three minutes.

Meanwhile, fry the mushrooms on a medium heat, keeping them moving in the pan until golden (approximately 3 minutes).

Use a slotted spoon to remove the egg from the water and drain on a piece of kitchen towel

Place the egg in the centre of the toast, surround with the mushrooms and serve immediately.

Lunch

Quick Bruschetta: 204 calories

84g (3 oz) tomatoes, chopped
14g (½ oz) red onion, finely chopped
½ small clove of garlic, crushed
1 tsp olive oil
Tiny sprinkle sugar – edge of tsp
3 large leaves fresh basil, chopped
1 thick slice of crusty bread
10ml (2 tsp) olive oil for the bread

Mix together all the ingredients except the bread and 10ml olive oil.

Drizzle 10ml olive oil on the bread.

Lightly toast bread on both sides under the grill.

Spread mixture evenly on toasted bread and serve.

Use knife and fork to eat.

Supper

Cauliflower Bake: 157 calories

1 small potato, cubed
3 oz (84g) cauliflower florets
3 cherry tomatoes

Sauce:
1 tsp butter
1 baby leek, chopped
½ small clove garlic, chopped
1 level tsp plain flour
60ml (2 fl.oz) almond milk
14g (½ oz) grated cheddar cheese
Small pinch paprika

Preheat oven to 350°F/175 °C/Gas Mark 5

Boil potato cubes in pan of water until cooked but firm.

Steam cauliflower until tender (about 4 minutes).

Sauce:

Melt butter in a pan, add leek and garlic and sauté for 1 minute.

Stir in the flour until smoothly blended.

Remove the pan from heat and slowly add the almond milk, stirring continuously.

Add cheese and paprika.

Put the cauliflower in small ovenproof dish with cherry tomatoes and cooked potatoes.

Stir in the sauce

Bake for about 12 minutes until thoroughly heated.

Day 2: 495 calories

Breakfast

Apple and walnut Porridge: 159 calories

10g (1/3 oz) porridge oats
10g (1/3 oz) raisins
10g (1/3 oz) chopped walnuts
60ml (2 fl.oz) pure apple juice

Mix all ingredients well in a microwaveable bowl.

Microwave for 1½ minutes (based on 700W – adjust time accordingly).

Stir and serve.

Lunch

Asparagus Omelette: 100 calories

> 1-cal olive oil spray
> 1 large egg
> 1 tsp finely chopped herbs, fresh
> Salt and ground black pepper
> 5 asparagus tips
> 3 cherry tomatoes, halved
> Sprig of parsley

Cook asparagus in a few inches of boiling water in a covered saucepan for about 8 minutes until the tips are tender.

Drain, return to pan and cover to keep warm.

Coat an omelette pan with 4 sprays of 1-cal olive oil and heat gently over medium heat.

Whisk egg.

Add herbs, salt and pepper to taste.

Pour mixture into pan and spread evenly.

When set, and golden on the underside, arrange asparagus on one side and fold omelette in half.

Slide onto warmed plate, garnish with parsley and decorate with tomatoes.

Supper

Stir Fry Bok Choy: 236 calories

> 112g (4 oz) firm tofu, drained
> ½ tbsp hulled sesame seeds
> 2 tsp toasted sesame oil, divided
> 170g (6 oz) large bok choy, chopped
> 28g (1 oz) cooked black beans
> 1 small clove garlic, minced
> ½ tbsp minced fresh ginger
> ½ tsp dark brown sugar
> ½ tbsp low-sodium tamari
> A few drops of chilli-garlic sauce

Cut tofu into small cubes.

Roll cubes in sesame seeds.

Heat 1 tsp sesame oil in a non-stick frying pan over a medium heat.

Add tofu, and cook until golden brown (approx. 10 min.), turning occasionally. Put to one side.

Heat remaining oil in a wok over high heat.

Stir-fry the bok choy for 4 minutes.

Add black beans, garlic and ginger and continue to stir-fry for a further 2 minutes.

Stir in brown sugar and tamari, then add chilli-garlic sauce

Fold in the tofu before serving.

Day 3: 495 calories

Breakfast

Apple and Cucumber Refresher: 60 calories

70ml (2½ fl.oz) pure apple juice
112g (4 oz) cucumber, peeled and chopped
5g fresh mint, chopped
5 ice cubes

Pour the apple juice into a blender.

Add the cucumber and mint and ice cubes.

Blend on a high setting until completely smooth.

Pour into a glass and serve immediately.

This is a refreshing start to a summer morning!

Lunch

Sweet and Savoury Salad: 240 calories

    1 small orange, segmented
    56 g (2 oz) strawberries, halved
    56 g (2 oz) mixed salad leaves
    10 g toasted pecan nuts

    Cinnamon & Ginger Vinaigrette:

    2 tsp olive oil
    2 tsp orange juice
    ¼ tsp ground ginger
    ¼ tsp ground cinnamon
    Stevia to taste
    Sea salt and black pepper to taste

Combine the salad ingredients in a bowl.

Make the vinaigrette, by mixing all its ingredients together well.

Pour the vinaigrette over the salad and toss the salad to ensure even coating.

Serve immediately.

Supper

Cheese & Onion Frittata: 195 calories

3 tablespoons "2 Chicks" liquid egg white*
30ml (2 tbsp) semi-skimmed milk
5ml (1 tsp) fresh parsley, chopped
Salt and freshly ground pepper to taste
1 small carrot, chopped
½ small onion, chopped
28g (1 oz) cheddar cheese, grated
1-cal olive oil spray

This quantity is based on "2 Chicks" Liquid Egg White and is equivalent to 1 egg. Other brands may vary.

Whisk together the egg white, milk, parsley, salt and pepper.

Coat a small omelette pan with 6 sprays of 1-cal olive oil spray and heat gently.

Fry the carrot and onion for a few minutes until tender.

Pour egg mixture over vegetables and sprinkle with cheese.

Cook on a low heat for approx. 5 minutes until the mixture has set and the underside is golden brown.

Transfer to a warmed plate for serving.

Day 4: 500 calories

Breakfast

Fruity Oatbars: 135 calories in 1 bar
(Makes 8, 1 to eat now, the rest to wrap and freeze)

> 84g (3 oz) rolled oats
> ½ tsp almond extract
> 2 tbsp honey
> 56g (2 oz) peanut butter
> 56g (2 oz) chopped almonds
> 28g (1 oz) flax seeds
> 1 tsp cinnamon
> ¼ tsp nutmeg
> 1 tsp vanilla extract
> ½ small banana

Combine all ingredients until well mixed.

Spread the mixture evenly into a small baking tin and press down well.

Place in freezer for approximately 1 hour, until firm.

Slice into 8 equal bars.

Foil-wrap all but one and freeze until required.

Lunch

Fresh Fruit Salad: 175 calories

28g (1 oz) blueberries
1 medium plum, stoned and chopped
1 satsuma, segmented
1 apricot, halved
1 small banana, sliced
84g (3 oz) strawberries, sliced
5 seedless grapes
Small wedge honeydew melon, cubed
Juice of 1 lemon, freshly squeezed
Stevia to taste

Combine all the fruit in a bowl.

Pour lemon juice over and mix well.

Sweeten with stevia as required.

Serve at room temperature or chill if preferred.

Supper

Scrambled Egg with Chives: 190 calories

2 small eggs
15ml (½ fl oz) skimmed milk
2g (½ tsp) butter
1 slice wholemeal bread
¼ tsp oregano
2 fresh chives, finely chopped
Sea salt and white pepper to season

Whisk eggs and milk vigorously.

Season with salt and pepper.

Toast bread on both sides.

Melt butter gently in saucepan over low heat.

Add egg mixture and increase heat to medium.

Stir until cooked to desired consistency.

Sprinkle with oregano and remove from heat.

Top the toast evenly with the egg.

Garnish with chives.

Day 5: 500 Calories

Breakfast

Hot Grain Breakfast: 188 calories

> 60ml (2 fl.oz) fat free milk
> 28g (1 oz) couscous
> 28g (2 oz) raisins
> 28g (1 oz) blueberries
> Stevia to taste

Microwave milk until hot (about 40 seconds or less, depending on your microwave).

Add couscous to milk and allow to stand for 5 minutes.

Stir in raisins and blueberries.

Add stevia to taste.

Lunch

Fruit & Ginger Smoothie: 128 calories

      1 passion fruit
      56g (2 oz) prepacked fresh or frozen mango slices
      1 extra small banana
      60ml (2 fl.oz) apple juice
      ½ tsp ground ginger
      Ice cubes (optional)

Cut passion fruit in half, scoop out the flesh and seeds and discard the shell.

Place all ingredients into a blender.

Blend thoroughly until smooth.

Add ice if desired and serve

Supper

Spinach & Onion Omelette: 184 calories

      1-cal olive oil
      2 tbsp chopped onion
      ½ tsp dried Italian seasoning
      28 g (1 oz) torn spinach leaves
      2 medium eggs
      Pinch ground black pepper
      2 tbsp (½ oz.) shredded part-skimmed mozzarella cheese

Coat an omelette pan with 6 sprays of olive oil over medium heat.

Add onion and Italian seasoning and fry until onion is tender (approx.3 min).

Add spinach leaves and cook briefly until they wilt (approx. 1 min).

Remove from heat and set mixture on a plate to one side.

Respray pan with 4 sprays of olive oil and place over medium heat.

Whisk the eggs and add pepper.

Pour the egg mixture into the pan and cook until it begins to set and the underside is golden brown.

Place the vegetable mixture and cheese on one half of the egg and fold the other half over.

Allow to cook for a further minute to allow the cheese to melt.

Slide onto a plate and serve while hot.

Day 6: 497 calories

Breakfast

Oatmeal & Blueberry Breakfast: 95 calories

10g ($^1/_3$ oz) porridge oats
Pinch of cinnamon
56g (2 oz) blueberries
60ml soya milk

Mix oats with cinnamon and soya milk.

Microwave for 1½ minutes (based on 700W – adjust accordingly).

Add blueberries and stir.

Microwave for 30 seconds.

Stir and serve.

Lunch

Miso Aubergines: 153 calories

>1 small aubergine, halved lengthways
>1-cal olive oil
>Sea salt
>Ground pepper
>1 tbsp miso paste
>1 tbsp apple juice
>Pinch of stevia
>½ tbsp lemon juice
>½ tbsp sesame seeds
>2 spring onions, chopped
>Rocket (arugula) leaves, small handful

Preheat oven to 200ºC/390ºF/Gas Mark 6.

Use a sharp knife to score the flesh of the aubergine halves with a criss-cross pattern.

Spray each half with 3 sprays of oil and season with salt and pepper.

Place on non stick baking tray and roast for 20 minutes.

Heat grill to high temperature.

Mix miso and apple juice with stevia and lemon juice.

Spread the mixture over cooked aubergines.

Sprinkle with sesame seeds.

Grill until golden, 2-3 minutes.

Serve on a bed of rocket leaves and garnished with spring onions.

Supper

Lemon and Parsley Couscous: 249 calories

60g (2 oz) couscous
210ml (7 fl.oz) vegetable stock, boiling
1 small tomato, chopped
28g (1 oz) pomegranate seeds
28g (1 oz) spring onions, finely sliced
Pinch garlic granules
Pinch dried chillies, crushed
½ tsp parsley, chopped
2 tsp lemon juice
2 tsp olive oil
28g (1 oz) light halloumi cheese
Sea salt
Black pepper

Place couscous in a pan or heatproof bowl and pour in the vegetable stock.

Add the remaining ingredients except lemon juice, olive oil and halloumi, salt and pepper.

Cover and put to one side for 10 minutes.

Slice halloumi.

Heat oil in non-stick frying pan and fry halloumi slices until golden on both sides.

Fluff couscous with a fork.

Drizzle couscous with lemon juice, add salt and pepper and toss lightly.

Serve with halloumi slices.

Day 7: 499 calories

Breakfast

Carrot and Mango Crush: 185 calories

28g (2 oz) prepacked fresh mango slices
75ml (2½ fl.oz) freshly-squeezed orange juice
30ml (1 fl.oz) carrot juice
Crushed ice, to serve
Rocket (arugula) leaves, to decorate

Place all ingredients, except ice and rocket, into a blender.

Blend until smooth.

Pour into tall glass, stir in ice and top with rocket leaves.

Lunch

Spicy Onion & Tomato Salad: 47 calories

    1 very small onion, sliced
    1 medium vine tomato, sliced
    ¼ green chilli, deseeded and finely chopped
    ½ tbsp lemon juice
    ¼ tsp coriander leaf, finely chopped
    Sea salt to taste

Mix together tomato and onion slices and chopped chilli.

Stir in lemon juice, coriander leaf and salt.

Refrigerate for approximately an hour and serve chilled.

Supper

Feta Tortilla Wrap: 267 calories

       1 10-inch whole-wheat tortilla
       42 g (1½ oz) feta cheese, crumbled
       2 black olives, sliced
       ¼ small yellow squash, sliced
       ¼ cucumber, diced
       4 cherry tomatoes, halved
       1 very small red onion, thinly sliced
       2 tsp balsamic vinegar
       ½ small clove garlic, minced
       2 tsp chopped fresh parsley
       ½ tsp olive oil
       Sea salt
       Black ground pepper

Mix all ingredients apart from tortilla in a bowl.

Allow to stand for 15 minutes, stirring occasionally.

Drain off liquid and place mixture on tortilla.

Fold bottom of wrap over lower part of filling.

Roll up the tortilla to form a wrap.

Day 8: 499 Calories

Breakfast

Spiced Fruit Smoothie: 192 calories

½ small banana, sliced
½ ripe pear, peeled and diced
1 small apple, peeled and diced
75ml (2½ fl.oz) apple juice
75ml (2½ fl.oz) low-fat vanilla yoghurt
Pinch of ground cinnamon
Mint leaves
Ice cubes

Place all ingredients, except mint and ice cubes, into a blender.

Whizz until smooth.

Pour into tall glass.

Add ice and top with mint leaves.

Lunch

Tomatoes with Okra & Onion: 71 calories

1-cal olive oil spray
1 small onion, chopped
½ clove garlic, crushed
Pinch cayenne pepper (go easy!)
½ green pepper, chopped
70g (2½ oz) okra, sliced
56g (2 oz) canned, chopped tomatoes with juice
1 fresh tomato, chopped
Sea salt
Ground black pepper

Coat frying pan with 6 sprays olive oil and heat over medium heat.

Add onion, garlic, green pepper, okra and cayenne pepper and cook until tender (approx. 4 minutes), stirring continuously.

Add canned tomatoes and juice and fresh tomato, season with salt and pepper.

Reduce heat to low and simmer until all vegetables are tender (approx. 4 minutes).

Supper

Vegetable Broth: 236 calories

2 tsp vegetable oil
1 small onion, chopped
1 tsp chopped rosemary
½ small garlic clove, chopped
1 small carrot, chopped
215ml vegetable stock
100g can chickpeas, drained
25g green beans, chopped

Heat the oil in a small pan over a medium heat.

Add onion, rosemary and garlic and fry for 2 minutes.

Add carrots and pour in stock.

Simmer for 10 minutes before mixing in the chickpeas.

Stir in the beans and simmer for a further 3 minutes.

Day 9: 500 calories

Breakfast

Blueberry-Packed Smoothie: 160 calories

> 120 ml (4 fl.oz) fat-free natural yoghurt
> 75 ml (2½ fl.oz) pure apple juice
> 150 g (5 oz) fresh blueberries
> Stevia to sweeten according to taste
> Ice as desired

Put yoghurt, apple juice and blueberries into a blender.

Blend until smooth.

Add stevia to taste and blend again briefly.

Add ice and pour into a tall glass.

Lunch

Edamame Salad: 127 calories

      56 g (2 oz) shelled edamame, fresh or frozen
      28 g (1 oz) thinly sliced red cabbage
      ½ small orange pepper, thinly sliced
      40g (1½ oz) finely diced pineapple
      10g golden raisins
      3g almonds, chopped
      1 tsp fresh mint, chopped
      1 tsp fresh lime juice
      1 tsp honey
      2 drops chile-garlic sauce

Boil edamame beans for 5 minutes (10 min. if frozen).

Drain and rinse with cold water.

Place edamame in a bowl and add the remaining ingredients.

Mix well before serving.

Supper

Chinese Ginger Vegetables: 213 calories

1-cal olive oil spray
½ inch fresh ginger, peeled & grated
1 small onion, sliced thinly
150g (5 oz) frozen mixed vegetables
56g (2 oz) fresh or frozen French beans, sliced
75ml (2½ fl.oz) water
1 tbsp dark brown sugar
1 tbsp cornflour
2 tbsp soy sauce
2 tbsp malt vinegar
½ tsp ground ginger

Coat large frying pan with 6 sprays of oil over medium heat.

Add ginger, fry for 1 minute.

Remove from pan and drain on piece of kitchen towelling and place to one side.

Place vegetables and water in the frying pan.

Cover, and cook for 5 – 6 minutes until vegetables are tender.

In a bowl, combine sugar, cornflour, soy sauce, malt vinegar and ground ginger.

Add this mix to the vegetables in the frying pan and simmer, whilst stirring, for 1 minute until liquid thickens.

Stir in the grated ginger.

Cook for a further two minutes before serving.

Day 10: 499 calories

Breakfast

Blueberry Quark Pancake: 130 calories

> 40g ((1½ oz) quark
> 3 tablespoons liquid egg-white*
> 100ml (3½ fl.oz) water
> 1 pinch salt
> 20g (¾ oz) plain flour
> 28g (1 oz) blueberries
> Stevia to taste
> 1-cal olive oil spray

This quantity is based on "2 Chicks" Liquid Egg White and is equivalent to 1 egg. Other brands may vary.

Whisk together quark, egg white, water, salt and flour.

Allow batter to stand for 10 minutes.

Coat small non-stick omelette pan with 4 sprays of 1-cal oil and heat on high temperature.

Reduce heat to medium and pour in batter to cover pan evenly.

Cook for approximately 3 minutes until almost set

Loosen edges with spatula and cook until the base is golden brown (1 – 2 minutes)

Sprinkle blueberries onto one half.

Add stevia to taste.

Fold carefully in half and slide onto warmed plate.

Lunch

Fresh Mediterranean Salad: 132 calories

6 Romaine lettuce leaves, torn
10 slices cucumber
½ small green pepper, sliced
2 cherry tomatoes, halved
½ very small onion, sliced into rings
2 radishes, thinly sliced
1 tsp fresh parsley, chopped

½ pita bread

Dressing:

7½ ml (1½ tsp) lemon juice
7½ ml (1½ tsp) olive oil
tiny piece garlic clove, crushed
2 mint leaves, finely chopped
sea salt
black pepper

Put all salad ingredients in a bowl and mix gently.

Thoroughly mix lemon juice, olive oil, garlic, mint, salt and pepper.

Pour dressing over salad and lightly toss to coat.

Serve with warmed pita bread.

Supper

Carrot & Lentil Soup: 237 calories

½ tsp cumin seeds
Very small pinch chilli flakes
½ tbsp olive oil
150g (5½ oz) grated carrot
35g (1½ oz) split red lentils
35 ml (1½ fl.oz) semi-skimmed or soya milk
250ml (8½ fl.oz) vegetable stock
1 tsp plain fat free yoghurt
5 coriander leaves, torn

Dry-fry cumin seeds and chilli flakes in a hot saucepan for approx 1 minute until you can smell the aroma.

Add oil, carrot, lentils, milk and vegetable stock and bring to the boil.

Reduce heat and simmer for 15 minutes until lentils are softened.

Serve, topped with yoghurt and coriander leaves.

Day 11: 500 calories

Breakfast

Orange Fruit Salad: 120 calories

1 large orange, peeled and cut horizontally into slices
40 ml (1½ fl.oz) orange juice
½ tsp mint, chopped
¼ tsp ground cinnamon
mint leaves to garnish

Mix together orange slices, orange juice and chopped mint in serving bowl.

Sprinkle with cinnamon.

Garnish with mint leaves.

Lunch

Red Pepper Soup: 77 calories

180ml (6 fl.oz) vegetable stock
½ red pepper
½ small onion
1 tiny clove garlic
1 small tomato, halved

Preheat oven to 180°C/350°F/Gas mark 4.

Place pepper, onion, garlic and tomato on a foil lined baking tray.

Roast for 10 minutes.

Remove skin from tomato and squeeze garlic from its skin.

Put all ingredients including stock in a blender and blend until smooth.

Pour into saucepan, heat gently and serve.

Supper

Stuffed Pepper: 303 calories

> 1 medium red pepper, cut in half, lengthways and deseeded
> 56g (2 oz) couscous
> 1-calorie olive oil spray
> 1 very small onion, chopped
> Juice and zest of ½ lemon
> 28g (1 oz) reduced fat feta cheese, crumbled
> ½ tsp ground coriander
> 1 dried apricot, chopped

Preheat oven to 200°C, 400°F, Gas Mark 6.

Place pepper halves on a baking tray (oiled or non-stick) and cook for 10 minutes until tender.

Meanwhile, cooking, pour 60 ml boiling water over the couscous, cover and leave for 10 minutes until absorbed.

Coat a small frying pan with 6 sprays of 1-calorie olive oil and heat gently.

Fry the onion, stirring constantly, for approx. 3 minutes until softened.

Add lemon juice and zest, feta cheese, coriander, apricot and onion to the couscous.

Stuff the roasted peppers with the couscous mixture and serve.

Day 12: 492 calories

Breakfast

Spiced Fruit Salad: 70 calories

56g (2 oz) melon
56g (2 oz) strawberries
56g (2 oz) grapes
56g (2 oz) apple slices
56g (2 oz) blackberries
¼ tsp mixed spice

Cut the melon into small chunks.

Slice the strawberries.

Halve the grapes.

Mix all fruit in a bowl with mixed spice.

Serve at room temperature or chilled.

Lunch

Summer Salad: 83 calories

70g cumber, peeled
2 medium tomatoes
20 g orange pepper
3 basil leaves
¼ clove garlic
1 tsp cider vinegar
½ tsp olive oil
sea salt
black pepper

Chop cucumber, tomatoes, pepper and basil into small pieces.

Mix with remainder of the ingredients and chill in refrigerator for 30 minutes.

Serve cold.

Supper

Twirly Pasta with Tomatoes, Spinach & Cheese: 339 calories

> 56g (2 oz) pasta twirls, cooked and drained
> ¾ tbsp olive oil
> ¾ tbsp white wine vinegar
> ¼ tsp thyme
> ¼ tsp rosemary
> pinch garlic granules
> pinch basil
> pinch oregano
> Sea salt to taste
> 14g (½ oz) baby spinach leaves
> 28g (1 oz) light mozzarella cheese, torn
> ½ tsp Parmesan-style vegetarian cheese, grated
> 56g (2 oz) cherry tomatoes, halved

Mix together oil, vinegar, thyme, rosemary, garlic, basil, oregano and sea salt.

Add cooked pasta and spinach and toss thoroughly.

Mix in cheeses and tomatoes.

Serve warm or allow to cool according to preference.

Day 13: 500 calories

Breakfast

Peanut Butter and Fruit Waffle: 165 calories

1 low fat waffle
½ tbsp peanut butter
½ small banana, sliced
2 strawberries, sliced

Toast the waffle on both sides.

Spread the peanut butter evenly on the waffle.

Decorate with alternate slices of banana and strawberries.

Lunch

Spicy Cauliflower: 140 calories

> 1-cal olive oil spray
> ¼ tsp cumin seeds
> ¼ small green chilli, chopped
> ¼ tsp chopped fresh ginger
> ½ tsp garlic pulp
> 120g (4 oz) cauliflower florets
> Pinch ground turmeric
> 28g (1 oz) peas
> Small pinch garam masala
> Small pinch ground cumin
> ½ tbsp fresh coriander, chopped
> 1 tsp lemon juice

Heat 10 sprays olive oil in a wok over a medium heat.

Put in cumin seeds, chilli, ginger and garlic and stir well.

Add cauliflower, turmeric and peas.

Sprinkle with a little water and cook for 10 minutes, stirring continuously.

When the cauliflower is tender but firm, stir in the garam masala, ground cumin, coriander and lemon juice and serve.

Supper

Basil & Tomato Scrambled Eggs: 195 calories

2 small eggs
1 tbsp onion, finely chopped
3 fresh basil leaves, finely chopped
4 cherry tomatoes, quartered
2 teaspoons Parmesan-style vegetarian cheese, grated
1 teaspoon butter
Salt & pepper to taste
2 crisp breads

Melt butter in a frying pan over low heat.

Turn heat to medium and sauté the onions for about 1 minute.

Add the eggs, basil, salt & pepper.

Cook for 1 to 2 minutes, stirring constantly to scramble.

Stir in tomatoes and cheese.

Remove from heat when eggs are thoroughly cooked.

Serve with a couple of crisp breads.

Day 14: 495 calories

Breakfast

Baked Spiced Grapefruit: 62 calories

½ medium grapefruit
1 teaspoon clear honey
¼ tsp ground cinnamon

Preheat oven to 190°C/375°F/Gas mark 5

Loosen grapefruit segments with a sharp fruit knife.

Drizzle with honey.

Sprinkle with cinnamon.

Bake for 15 minutes.

Serve hot

Lunch

Mediterranean Vegetable Roast: 91 calories

¼ red pepper, cut in chunks
¼ orange pepper, cut in chunks
½ courgette (zucchini), thickly sliced
½ red onion, sliced
½ tbsp olive oil
½ tsp mixed herbs

Preheat oven to 220°C, 425°F, Gas Mark 7.

Put red and orange peppers, courgette and onions into a small roasting tin.

Pour on olive oil and mix thoroughly to coat vegetables.

Roast for 30 minutes.

Sprinkle with mixed herbs and serve.

Supper

Spaghetti with Courgette (Zucchini) & Onion: 342 calories

    1-cal olive oil spray
    ½ medium onion, thickly sliced
    1 medium courgette, thickly sliced
    ½ tsp ground black pepper
    70g (2½ oz) dry spaghetti
    1½ tablespoons Parmesan-style vegetarian cheese
    6 large leaves from round lettuce

Cook spaghetti according to instructions on the packet.

Spray frying pan with 8 sprays of 1-cal oil over a medium heat.

Stir-fry onions and courgette slices, seasoned with pepper, for 6-8 minutes until tender.

Remove from heat.

Drain spaghetti, rinse with boiling water and transfer to bowl.

Add vegetables to spaghetti and mix well.

Arrange lettuce leaves on a plate and spoon the mixture onto the bed of leaves.

Sprinkle with cheese and serve.

Day 15: 500 calories

Breakfast

Spiced oranges: 100 calories

    2 navel (small) oranges
    1 tbsp lemon juice
    1 tbsp orange juice
    Large pinch ground cinnamon
    Stevia to suit your tastebuds

Use a sharp knife to remove the rind and pith from the oranges.

Divide the oranges into segments and arrange in a serving bowl.

Put the lemon juice, orange juice, cinnamon and stevia in a cup and mix thoroughly.

Pour over oranges before eating.

Lunch

Cauliflower Soup: 87 calories

240 ml (8 fl.oz) low sodium vegetable stock
1 tbsp lemon juice
Florets of ½ medium cauliflower
½ tbsp olive oil
1 tbsp spring onion, chopped
Pinch nutmeg
¼ tsp ground black pepper

Boil stock and lemon juice in saucepan.

Reduce heat to medium and add cauliflower.

Cook for approx. 10 minutes until tender.

Warm oil over medium heat in a non-stick frying pan.

Fry spring onion gently for approx. 5 minutes.

Add spring onion to cauliflower and stir well.

Use a hand blender to puree the solids or use a food processor to blend.

Stir in nutmeg and pepper, and serve.

Supper

Mixed Roast Vegetables with Pasta: 313 calories

1 small red pepper cut in chunks
112g (4 oz) fresh mushrooms
1 small onion cut in wedges
1 baby courgette (zucchini) cut in chunks
2 tsp olive oil
¼ teaspoon minced garlic
Sea salt to taste
Ground black pepper to taste
56g (2 oz) pasta

Preheat oven to 220°C, 425°F, Gas Mark 7.

Mix mushrooms, onion and courgette with olive oil, garlic and seasoning.

Spread onto a foil-lined oven tray.

Roast for approx. 15 minutes until tender.

Meanwhile, cook pasta according to instructions on package.

Rinse pasta with boiling water and drain.

Transfer to serving bowl and stir in the vegetable mixture.

Serve hot.

Day 16: 499 calories

Breakfast

Cheesy Toasty Breakfast: 99 calories

1 small slice wholemeal bread
28 g (1 oz) cottage cheese
1 tsp cinnamon
1 pineapple ring

Preheat grill to medium heat.

Toast bread on one side.

Spread cottage cheese evenly on untoasted side.

Sprinkle with cinnamon.

Top with pineapple ring.

Grill until cheese begins to brown.

Serve hot.

Lunch

Sweet & Sour Salad: 87 calories

     56g (2 oz) cauliflower
     3 tbsp fresh parsley, chopped
     10 cherry tomatoes
     2 g (1 oz) low fat yogurt
     30ml (1 fl oz) lemon juice

Cook the cauliflower until tender but firm and leave to cool.

Put the tomatoes and parsley in a bowl.

Add the cauliflower.

Mix together yogurt and lemon.

Spoon onto vegetables and mix well before serving.

Supper

Vegetable Goulash: 313 calories

    1-cal olive oil
    ¼ medium onion, thinly sliced
    56g (2 oz) Quorn pieces
    1 small green pepper, thinly sliced
    ½ teaspoon paprika
    ½ clove garlic, chopped
    200g (7 oz) canned chopped tomatoes with juice
    ½ teaspoon dried oregano
    ½ teaspoon tomato puree
    60ml (2 fl.oz) red wine
    Pinch stevia
    Sea salt
    Ground black pepper

Coat frying pan with 8 sprays olive oil over medium heat.

Fry onion until tender, then add Quorn and green pepper.

Cook for further 5 minutes, stirring continuously until pepper is tender.

Stir in paprika and garlic.

Add tomatoes and juice and stir well.

Mix in oregano and tomato puree and stir in wine.

Bring to boil, reduce heat, cover and simmer for 20 minutes, stirring occasionally.

When liquid is thickened, stir in stevia, salt and pepper.

Serve immediately.

Day 17: 494 calories

Breakfast

Pear and Ginger Smoothie: 190 calories

2 oranges
1 soft, juicy pear
1 tsp clear honey
1 small piece of ginger root (according to taste), finely
chopped

Preheat the grill to medium.

Cut the pear in half, removing core and stalk.

Place the halves flesh side up on a baking tray.

Brush with honey.

Heat for about 7 minutes until the flesh is softened and the honey
caramelises.

Squeeze the oranges and put the juice in a blender.

Add the pears and blend thoroughly.

Pour into a glass to serve.

Lunch

Coleslaw: 79 calories

28g (1 oz) cabbage, finely shredded
½ medium apple, cored and finely chopped
28g (1 oz) carrot, grated
1 tbsp Dijon mustard
2 tbsp extra light mayonnaise
1 tsp sugar
2 tsp lemon juice
½ tsp cumin
1 sprig parsley

Combine all ingredients except parsley in a bowl and mix thoroughly.

Garnish with parsley.

Supper

Chinese Ginger Vegetables: 225 calories

> 1-cal olive oil spray
> ½ inch fresh ginger, peeled & grated
> 1 small onion, sliced thinly
> 140g (5 oz) frozen mixed vegetables
> 84g (3 oz) fresh or frozen French beans, sliced
> 75ml (2½ fl.oz) water
> 1 tbsp dark brown sugar
> 1 tbsp cornflour
> 2 tbsp soy sauce
> 2 tbsp malt vinegar
> ½ tsp ground ginger

Coat large frying pan with 6 sprays of oil over medium heat.

Add ginger, fry for 1 minute.

Remove from pan and drain on piece of kitchen towelling and place to one side.

Place vegetables and water in the frying pan.

Cover, and cook for 5 – 6 minutes until vegetables are tender.

In a bowl, combine sugar, cornflour, soy sauce, malt vinegar and ground ginger.

Add this mix to the vegetables in the frying pan and simmer, whilst stirring, for 1 minute until liquid thickens.

Stir in the grated ginger.

Cook for a further two minutes before serving.

Day 18: 492 calories

Breakfast

Cucumber, Mint & Orange Refresher: 105 calories

½ small cucumber
1 tbsp fresh mint leaves
100ml (3½) fl.oz apple juice
10 ml (3½) freshly squeezed orange juice

Peel and cut cucumber into chunks.

Put cucumber and mint into a blender with apple and orange juice.

Whizz thoroughly until smooth.

Pour into a tall glass.

Lunch

Quick Minestrone Soup: 197 calories

> 2 medium tomatoes
> 28g 1 oz) dry spaghetti
> 250ml (8 fl.oz) vegetable stock
> 28g (1 oz) frozen peas
> 28g (1 oz) frozen peppers
> Sea salt
> Ground pepper

Place tomatoes in boiling water for a couple of minutes to loosen skin.

Remove skin and chop tomatoes.

Break spaghetti into small pieces and add to stock.

Boil stock and add tomato chunks.

Simmer gently for 5 minutes and season.

Add frozen vegetables and return to boil.

Simmer for further 2 minutes until vegetables are tender.

Pour into bowl and serve.

Supper

Pasta with Tomato Sauce: 190 calories

28g (1 oz) penne pasta
1-cal olive oil spray
1 clove garlic, crushed
½ small onion, chopped
28g (1 oz) celery, chopped
20g mushrooms, sliced
1 tablespoon grated carrot, grated
1 small basil leaf, finely chopped
¼ tbsp fresh thyme, finely chopped
200g canned, chopped tomatoes
Ground black pepper
Salt

Put a saucepan of lightly salted water to boil for the pasta.

Coat medium saucepan with 8 sprays olive oil.

Sauté garlic, onion, celery and mushrooms for about 5 minutes whilst stirring, until softened.

Add carrot, basil and thyme.

Cook for a further 5 minutes.

Pour in tomatoes with juice and bring to boil.

Reduce heat to low and season with pepper.

Cover and simmer for about 15 minutes, stirring occasionally.

Meanwhile, add pasta to boiling water and cook according to instructions on packet.

Drain pasta, rinse with boiling water and transfer to plate.

Pour mixture over pasta and serve immediately.

Day 19: 493 calories

Breakfast

Fresh Fruit and Vegetable juice: 145 calories

  1 apple
½ small lemon, peeled
 3 stalks celery
1 large carrot
227g (8 oz) spinach
Crushed ice

Put fruit and vegetables through the juicer

Place crushed ice into glass

Pour juice over and serve

Lunch

Carrot and Cumin Soup: 108 calories
(Delicious hot or cold)

> 1-calorie olive oil spray
> 1 clove garlic, crushed
> 1 baby leek, chopped,
> 1 tbsp onion, chopped
> ½ tsp cumin
> Pinch cayenne pepper
> 120ml (4fl.oz) vegetable stock
> 1 large carrot, chopped
> Ground black pepper

Coat a saucepan with 8 sprays of oil and heat gently.

Add garlic, leek and onion and cook for approx 4 minutes until vegetables soften

Turn heat to medium pour in stock and add cumin, cayenne pepper and stock.

Bring to boil and add carrots.

Simmer for 15 minutes or until carrots are tender

Puree mixture in a blender until smooth

Add ground pepper to taste

Supper

Tofu and Quinoa: 240 calories

90ml (3fl. oz) water
Pinch of salt
42g (1½ oz) quinoa
1 tbsp lemon juice
½ tbsp virgin olive oil
½ clove garlic, minced
Pinch of black ground pepper
42g (1½ oz) baked smoked tofu, diced
¼ yellow pepper, diced
2 cherry tomatoes, halved
42g (1½ oz) cucumber, diced
1 tbsp fresh parsley, chopped
1 tbsp fresh mint, chopped

Add quinoa to boiling, salted water.

Reduce to simmer, cover and cook until all water is absorbed (10 - 15 minutes).

Spread out quinoa on a baking tray to cool for approx. 10 minutes.

While it is cooling, whisk lemon juice, oil, garlic, salt and pepper.

Add quinoa, tofu, pepper, tomatoes, cucumber, parsley and mint.

Toss well before serving.

Day 20: 500 calories

Breakfast

Spicy Apple and Kiwi Smoothie: 80 calories

1 small Granny Smith apple, cored and sliced
½ kiwi fruit, peeled
1 small celery stalk
42g (1½ oz) parsley leaves
½ tbsp fresh ginger, minced
1 tsp lime juice

Place all ingredients apart from lime juice into juice extractor.

Stir in lime juice, pour into a glass and serve.

Lunch

Yoghurt Waldorf Salad: 233 calories

58g (2 oz) celery sticks, thinly sliced
1 small red eating apple, cored and sliced
14g (½ oz) chopped walnuts,
14g (½ oz) raisins
56g (2 oz) natural low-fat yoghurt
½ tbsp lemon juice
4 leaves from round lettuce
Sea salt & ground black pepper to season

Thoroughly mix yoghurt and lemon juice.

Add salt and pepper.

Stir in celery, apple, walnuts and raisins.

Refrigerate for approximately one hour.

Serve chilled on a bed of lettuce.

Supper

Spiced Lentil Stew: 187 calories

50g lentils
120 ml (4 fl.oz) water
½ small onion, chopped
1 celery stalk, chopped
70g (2½ oz) canned chopped tomatoes
1½ cloves garlic, crushed
Small sprinkle curry powder (to taste)
Sea salt
Ground black pepper

Put lentils in water and bring to boil.

Turn heat to simmer and add onion, celery, tomatoes and garlic.

Cover and simmer for 35 minutes, stirring occasionally and adding more water if required.

Add curry powder, salt and pepper halfway through cooking.

Printed in Great Britain
by Amazon.co.uk, Ltd.,
Marston Gate.